One Hour Gym

30 Day Workout

By Mark F Kalita

To connect with the author, please visit:
www.OneHourGym.com

Individual exercises will not be discussed or demonstrated, but merely listed within this book, "One Hour Gym: 30 Day Workout".

As this book, "One Hour Gym: 30 Day Workout", is based on the assumption that users of this book will have a gym membership, guidelines for usage and safety for this equipment is part of your gym membership. If you do not understand how to use a particular piece of equipment safely at your gym, please ask gym personnel for assistance before starting any exercise within "One Hour Gym: 30 Day Workout".

The creators of "One Hour Gym: 30 Day Workout" are not responsible for a participant's usage of equipment in connection with completing the exercises contained within "One Hour Gym: 30 Day Workout".

Consult a physician before starting any fitness program.

Dedicated to ALL!
Get Healthy!
Get Fit!
One hour at a time with the
One Hour Gym!

Table of Contents

Forward

One Hour Gym

This is your "One Hour Gym: 30 Day Workout". Take it with you. Write in it. Learn the program. Track your progress. Find a friendly workout buddy. Share your success. Work together. Motivate each other.

The "One Hour Gym" is actually a 30 day fitness program revolving around a set of standard muscle strength and definition exercises to maximize your time in the gym. These exercises utilize common equipment found in gyms around the world. Using a combination of weights and machines, the "One Hour Gym" workout simplifies the science of building muscle for strength and definition.

By utilizing the sets of exercises found within the "One Hour Gym" workout, muscle strength and definition is virtually guaranteed based upon the science of fitness. "One Hour Gym" actually incorporates decades old standards to building muscle mass with a new system of measurement and quantitative results that have been shown to maximize muscle gains. All of this while working out only ONE HOUR per day in any gym worldwide.

Bottom line – **Work "One Hour Gym" for results!**

Chapter 1
Evaluate

The "One Hour Gym: 30 Day Workout" is a series of 9 exercises per day for 6 days. These exercises work the entire body over the course of 6 days. One day of the week is used for muscle recovery.

At the beginning of a 30 day "One Hour Gym" cycle, the participant is required to do one exercise in determining the weight measures used throughout this workout program – Maximum Machine Bench Press.

Once the participant's 'Maximum Machine Bench Press' weight is discovered, the starting weights for this 30 day "One Hour Gym" workout cycle can be determined.

The formulas for approximating starting weights within the "One Hour Gym" workout program are:

Bench Press X .2 = Arm Dumbbell Weight
Bench Press X .3 = Chest Dumbbell Weight
Bench Press X .4 = Back Dumbbell Weights
Bench Press X .5 = Cable Weight
Bench Press X 1.2 = Leg Weights

Date: _____ Machine Bench Press(BP) _____lbs

BP X .2 = Arm Dumbbell Weight _____lbs

BP X .3 = Chest Dumbbell Weight _____lbs

BP X .4 = Back Dumbbell Weights _____lbs

BP X .5 = Cable Weight _____lbs

BP X 1.2 = Leg Weights _____lbs

Date: _____ Machine Bench Press(BP) _____lbs

BP X .2 = Arm Dumbbell Weight _____lbs

BP X .3 = Chest Dumbbell Weight _____lbs

BP X .4 = Back Dumbbell Weights _____lbs

BP X .5 = Cable Weight _____lbs

BP X 1.2 = Leg Weights _____lbs

Date: _____ Machine Bench Press(BP) _____lbs

BP X .2 = Arm Dumbbell Weight _____lbs

BP X .3 = Chest Dumbbell Weight _____lbs

BP X .4 = Back Dumbbell Weights _____lbs

BP X .5 = Cable Weight _____lbs

BP X 1.2 = Leg Weights _____lbs

Date: _____ Machine Bench Press(BP) _____lbs

BP X .2 = Arm Dumbbell Weight _____lbs

BP X .3 = Chest Dumbbell Weight _____lbs

BP X .4 = Back Dumbbell Weights _____lbs

BP X .5 = Cable Weight _____lbs

BP X 1.2 = Leg Weights _____lbs

Date: _____ Machine Bench Press(BP) _____lbs

BP X .2 = Arm Dumbbell Weight _____lbs

BP X .3 = Chest Dumbbell Weight _____lbs

BP X .4 = Back Dumbbell Weights _____lbs

BP X .5 = Cable Weight _____lbs

Chapter 2
Goal

The 'Goal' of the "One Hour Gym: 30 Day Workout" is to complete one 30 day cycle of these muscle strengthening exercises.

By completing one 30 day cycle of these muscle strengthening exercises, participants should see verifiable gains in both muscle mass and strength. The most significant gains are reported by repeating the "One Hour Gym: 30 Day Workout" in succession. After 90 days, or only 3 "One Hour Gym" cycles, participants show significant muscle gains.

Individual goals within any single 30 day cycle may vary. An individual goal may be to do weekly individual muscle group concentrated exercises. At the end of the 6 days of exercises, there are 5 individual muscle group 'Extra Hour' workouts. Included are exercises targeting the Abs, Chest, Legs, Back and Arms.

If your goals are significant muscle mass or definition within any of these 'Extra Hour' concentrations, just do an extra hour on the days that this muscle group is highlighted. If a particular concentration is not exercised in a day, do not use that 'Extra Hour' concentration.

For example, on 'Day 4' the exercises work the abs, shoulders and triceps. Only do the 'Extra Hours' for 'Abs' on Day 4. On 'Day 6' the exercises work the abs, triceps and chest. On 'Day 6', you can do the 'Extra Hour' for Abs and Chest. Do not do any 'Extra Hour' exercises unless they are listed for that day and you will have maximum results.

Chapter 3
Work It

All of the exercises within "One Hour Gym: 30 Day Workout" utilize common equipment found within a membership gym. This guide was written specifically to assist participants who have gym memberships make the most of their time at the gym. "One Hour Gym" provides the full body workout for maximizing strength and definition of your muscles.

Each day, for 6 consecutive days, there is a series of 9 exercises. These 9 exercises are actually 3 each of 3 body groups per day. Each series takes less than 60 minutes to complete.

In addition to the 54 individual daily exercises, also included in "One Hour Gym: 30 Day Workout" are 5 specialized 'PUMP' exercise series to maximize the Abs, Arms, Chest, Legs or Back.

In the individual exercise logs, the abbreviations 'S1', 'S2' and 'S3' are 'Set 1', 'Set 2' and Set 3' respectively. Within each set, participants are to do 8 reps (repetitions) of the weight listed under '____ lbs'. Three sets of these 8 weight repetitions are a complete exercise. By keeping track of the weights, participants discover strength gains by continuing these exercises.

Chapter 4
Day 1

Day 1 of the "One Hour Gym" workout builds muscle mass and strength in the legs, back and chest.

Utilizing a set of 9 exercises, these three muscle groups will be worked to develop muscle mass and strength.

This series of exercises should take you less than 60 minutes to complete.

Dip Machine – Do all exercises 3 sets of 8 reps. Rest 60 seconds between sets. Rest 90 seconds after completing this exercise.

Date: _____ S1 _____ lbs S2 _____lbs S3 ____lbs

Date: _____ S1 _____ lbs S2 _____lbs S3 ____lbs

Date: _____ S1 _____ lbs S2 _____lbs S3 ____lbs

Date: _____ S1 _____ lbs S2 _____lbs S3 ____lbs

Date: _____ S1 _____ lbs S2 _____lbs S3 ____lbs

Leg Raise Machine – Do all exercises 3 sets of 8 reps. Rest 60 seconds between sets. Rest 90 seconds after completing this exercise.

Date: _____ S1 _____ lbs S2 _____lbs S3 ____lbs

Date: _____ S1 _____ lbs S2 _____lbs S3 ____lbs

Date: _____ S1 _____ lbs S2 _____lbs S3 ____lbs

Date: _____ S1 _____ lbs S2 _____lbs S3 ____lbs

Date: _____ S1 _____ lbs S2 _____lbs S3 ____lbs

Cable Lat Pull-down, Norman Overhand Grip – Do all exercises 3 sets of 8 reps. Rest 60 seconds between sets. Rest 90 seconds after completing this exercise.

Date: _____ S1 _____ lbs S2 _____lbs S3 ____lbs

Date: _____ S1 _____ lbs S2 _____lbs S3 ____lbs

Date: _____ S1 _____ lbs S2 _____lbs S3 ____lbs

Date: _____ S1 _____ lbs S2 _____lbs S3 ____lbs

Date: _____ S1 _____ lbs S2 _____lbs S3 ____lbs

Dumbbell Bench Press, Normal Grip – Do all exercises 3 sets of 8 reps. Rest 60 seconds between sets. Rest 90 seconds after completing this exercise.

Date: _____ S1 _____ lbs S2 _____lbs S3 ____lbs

Date: _____ S1 _____ lbs S2 _____lbs S3 ____lbs

Date: _____ S1 _____ lbs S2 _____lbs S3 ____lbs

Date: _____ S1 _____ lbs S2 _____lbs S3 ____lbs

Date: _____ S1 _____ lbs S2 _____lbs S3 ____lbs

Abduction Machine – Do all exercises 3 sets of 8 reps. Rest 60 seconds between sets. Rest 90 seconds after completing this exercise.

Date: _____ S1 _____ lbs S2 _____lbs S3 ____lbs

Date: _____ S1 _____ lbs S2 _____lbs S3 ____lbs

Date: _____ S1 _____ lbs S2 _____lbs S3 ____lbs

Date: _____ S1 _____ lbs S2 _____lbs S3 ____lbs

Date: _____ S1 _____ lbs S2 _____lbs S3 ____lbs

Cable Lat Pull-down Leaning Back, Wide Overhand Grip – Do all exercises 3 sets of 8 reps. Rest 60 seconds between sets. Rest 90 seconds after completing this exercise.

Date: _____ S1 _____ lbs S2 _____lbs S3 ____lbs

Date: _____ S1 _____ lbs S2 _____lbs S3 ____lbs

Date: _____ S1 _____ lbs S2 _____lbs S3 ____lbs

Date: _____ S1 _____ lbs S2 _____lbs S3 ____lbs

Date: _____ S1 _____ lbs S2 _____lbs S3 ____lbs

Dumbbell Fly – Do all exercises 3 sets of 8 reps. Rest 60 seconds between sets. Rest 90 seconds after completing this exercise.

Date: _____ S1 _____ lbs S2 _____lbs S3 ____lbs

Date: _____ S1 _____ lbs S2 _____lbs S3 ____lbs

Date: _____ S1 _____ lbs S2 _____lbs S3 ____lbs

Date: _____ S1 _____ lbs S2 _____lbs S3 ____lbs

Date: _____ S1 _____ lbs S2 _____lbs S3 ____lbs

Calf Press Machine – Do all exercises 3 sets of 8 reps. Rest 60 seconds between sets. Rest 90 seconds after completing this exercise.

Date: _____ S1 _____ lbs S2 _____lbs S3 ____lbs

Date: _____ S1 _____ lbs S2 _____lbs S3 ____lbs

Date: _____ S1 _____ lbs S2 _____lbs S3 ____lbs

Date: _____ S1 _____ lbs S2 _____lbs S3 ____lbs

Date: _____ S1 _____ lbs S2 _____lbs S3 ____lbs

Dumbbell Shrug, Incline Bench – Do all exercises 3 sets of 8 reps. Rest 60 seconds between sets. Rest 90 seconds after completing this exercise.

Date: _____ S1 _____ lbs S2 _____lbs S3 ____lbs

Date: _____ S1 _____ lbs S2 _____lbs S3 ____lbs

Date: _____ S1 _____ lbs S2 _____lbs S3 ____lbs

Date: _____ S1 _____ lbs S2 _____lbs S3 ____lbs

Date: _____ S1 _____ lbs S2 _____lbs S3 ____lbs

Chapter 5
Day 2

Day 2 of the "One Hour Gym" workout builds muscle mass and strength in the abs, arms and shoulders.

Utilizing a set of 9 exercises, these three muscle groups will be worked to develop muscle mass and strength.

This series of exercises should take you less than 60 minutes to complete.

Ab Machine – Do all exercises 3 sets of 8 reps. Rest 60 seconds between sets. Rest 90 seconds after completing this exercise.

Date: _____ S1 _____ lbs S2 _____lbs S3 ____lbs

Date: _____ S1 _____ lbs S2 _____lbs S3 ____lbs

Date: _____ S1 _____ lbs S2 _____lbs S3 ____lbs

Date: _____ S1 _____ lbs S2 _____lbs S3 ____lbs

Date: _____ S1 _____ lbs S2 _____lbs S3 ____lbs

Biceps Curl Machine – Do all exercises 3 sets of 8 reps. Rest 60 seconds between sets. Rest 90 seconds after completing this exercise.

Date: _____ S1 _____ lbs S2 _____lbs S3 ____lbs

Date: _____ S1 _____ lbs S2 _____lbs S3 ____lbs

Date: _____ S1 _____ lbs S2 _____lbs S3 ____lbs

Date: _____ S1 _____ lbs S2 _____lbs S3 ____lbs

Date: _____ S1 _____ lbs S2 _____lbs S3 ____lbs

Shoulder Press Machine – Do all exercises 3 sets of 8 reps. Rest 60 seconds between sets. Rest 90 seconds after completing this exercise.

Date: _____ S1 _____ lbs S2 _____lbs S3 ____lbs

Date: _____ S1 _____ lbs S2 _____lbs S3 ____lbs

Date: _____ S1 _____ lbs S2 _____lbs S3 ____lbs

Date: _____ S1 _____ lbs S2 _____lbs S3 ____lbs

Date: _____ S1 _____ lbs S2 _____lbs S3 ____lbs

Dumbbell Side Bend – Do all exercises 3 sets of 8 reps. Rest 60 seconds between sets. Rest 90 seconds after completing this exercise.

Date: _____ S1 _____ lbs S2 _____lbs S3 ____lbs

Date: _____ S1 _____ lbs S2 _____lbs S3 ____lbs

Date: _____ S1 _____ lbs S2 _____lbs S3 ____lbs

Date: _____ S1 _____ lbs S2 _____lbs S3 ____lbs

Date: _____ S1 _____ lbs S2 _____lbs S3 ____lbs

Dumbbell Biceps Curl, On Knee, Underhand Grip – Do all exercises 3 sets of 8 reps. Rest 60 seconds between sets. Rest 90 seconds after completing this exercise.

Date: _____ S1 _____ lbs S2 _____lbs S3 ____lbs

Date: _____ S1 _____ lbs S2 _____lbs S3 ____lbs

Date: _____ S1 _____ lbs S2 _____lbs S3 ____lbs

Date: _____ S1 _____ lbs S2 _____lbs S3 ____lbs

Date: _____ S1 _____ lbs S2 _____lbs S3 ____lbs

Dumbbell Front Raise – Do all exercises 3 sets of 8 reps. Rest 60 seconds between sets. Rest 90 seconds after completing this exercise.

Date: _____ S1 _____ lbs S2 _____lbs S3 ____lbs

Date: _____ S1 _____ lbs S2 _____lbs S3 ____lbs

Date: _____ S1 _____ lbs S2 _____lbs S3 ____lbs

Date: _____ S1 _____ lbs S2 _____lbs S3 ____lbs

Date: _____ S1 _____ lbs S2 _____lbs S3 ____lbs

Weighted Situps – Do all exercises 3 sets of 8 reps. Rest 60 seconds between sets. Rest 90 seconds after completing this exercise.

Date: _____ S1 _____ lbs S2 _____lbs S3 ____lbs

Date: _____ S1 _____ lbs S2 _____lbs S3 ____lbs

Date: _____ S1 _____ lbs S2 _____lbs S3 ____lbs

Date: _____ S1 _____ lbs S2 _____lbs S3 ____lbs

Date: _____ S1 _____ lbs S2 _____lbs S3 ____lbs

Dumbbell Biceps Curl, Incline, Alternating Overhead Grip – Do all exercises 3 sets of 8 reps. Rest 60 seconds between sets. Rest 90 seconds after completing this exercise.

Date: _____ S1 _____ lbs S2 _____lbs S3 ____lbs

Date: _____ S1 _____ lbs S2 _____lbs S3 ____lbs

Date: _____ S1 _____ lbs S2 _____lbs S3 ____lbs

Date: _____ S1 _____ lbs S2 _____lbs S3 ____lbs

Date: _____ S1 _____ lbs S2 _____lbs S3 ____lbs

Upright Cable Row – Do all exercises 3 sets of 8 reps. Rest 60 seconds between sets. Rest 90 seconds after completing this exercise.

Date: _____ S1 _____ lbs S2 _____lbs S3 ____lbs

Date: _____ S1 _____ lbs S2 _____lbs S3 ____lbs

Date: _____ S1 _____ lbs S2 _____lbs S3 ____lbs

Date: _____ S1 _____ lbs S2 _____lbs S3 ____lbs

Date: _____ S1 _____ lbs S2 _____lbs S3 ____lbs

Chapter 6
Day 3

Day 3 of the "One Hour Gym" workout builds muscle mass and strength in the legs, chest and back.

Utilizing a set of 9 exercises, these three muscle groups will be worked to develop muscle mass and strength.

This series of exercises should take you less than 60 minutes to complete.

Hamstring Pullback Machine – Do all exercises 3 sets of 8 reps. Rest 60 seconds between sets. Rest 90 seconds after completing this exercise.

Date: _____ S1 _____ lbs S2 _____lbs S3 ____lbs

Date: _____ S1 _____ lbs S2 _____lbs S3 ____lbs

Date: _____ S1 _____ lbs S2 _____lbs S3 ____lbs

Date: _____ S1 _____ lbs S2 _____lbs S3 ____lbs

Date: _____ S1 _____ lbs S2 _____lbs S3 ____lbs

Incline Dumbbell Fly – Do all exercises 3 sets of 8 reps. Rest 60 seconds between sets. Rest 90 seconds after completing this exercise.

Date: _____ S1 _____ lbs S2 _____lbs S3 ____lbs

Date: _____ S1 _____ lbs S2 _____lbs S3 ____lbs

Date: _____ S1 _____ lbs S2 _____lbs S3 ____lbs

Date: _____ S1 _____ lbs S2 _____lbs S3 ____lbs

Date: _____ S1 _____ lbs S2 _____lbs S3 ____lbs

Dumbbell Row, Single Arm, Neutral Grip – Do all exercises 3 sets of 8 reps. Rest 60 seconds between sets. Rest 90 seconds after completing this exercise.

Date: _____ S1 _____ lbs S2 _____lbs S3 ____lbs

Date: _____ S1 _____ lbs S2 _____lbs S3 ____lbs

Date: _____ S1 _____ lbs S2 _____lbs S3 ____lbs

Date: _____ S1 _____ lbs S2 _____lbs S3 ____lbs

Date: _____ S1 _____ lbs S2 _____lbs S3 ____lbs

Leg Raise Machine – Do all exercises 3 sets of 8 reps. Rest 60 seconds between sets. Rest 90 seconds after completing this exercise.

Date: _____ S1 _____ lbs S2 _____lbs S3 ____lbs

Date: _____ S1 _____ lbs S2 _____lbs S3 ____lbs

Date: _____ S1 _____ lbs S2 _____lbs S3 ____lbs

Date: _____ S1 _____ lbs S2 _____lbs S3 ____lbs

Date: _____ S1 _____ lbs S2 _____lbs S3 ____lbs

Chest Press Machine – Do all exercises 3 sets of 8 reps. Rest 60 seconds between sets. Rest 90 seconds after completing this exercise.

Date: _____ S1 _____ lbs S2 _____lbs S3 ____lbs

Date: _____ S1 _____ lbs S2 _____lbs S3 ____lbs

Date: _____ S1 _____ lbs S2 _____lbs S3 ____lbs

Date: _____ S1 _____ lbs S2 _____lbs S3 ____lbs

Date: _____ S1 _____ lbs S2 _____lbs S3 ____lbs

Cable Lat Pull-down Leaning Back, Narrow Overhand Grip – Do all exercises 3 sets of 8 reps. Rest 60 seconds between sets. Rest 90 seconds after completing this exercise.

Date: _____ S1 _____ lbs S2 _____lbs S3 ____lbs

Date: _____ S1 _____ lbs S2 _____lbs S3 ____lbs

Date: _____ S1 _____ lbs S2 _____lbs S3 ____lbs

Date: _____ S1 _____ lbs S2 _____lbs S3 ____lbs

Date: _____ S1 _____ lbs S2 _____lbs S3 ____lbs

Abduction Machine – Do all exercises 3 sets of 8 reps. Rest 60 seconds between sets. Rest 90 seconds after completing this exercise.

Date: _____ S1 _____ lbs S2 _____lbs S3 ____lbs

Date: _____ S1 _____ lbs S2 _____lbs S3 ____lbs

Date: _____ S1 _____ lbs S2 _____lbs S3 ____lbs

Date: _____ S1 _____ lbs S2 _____lbs S3 ____lbs

Date: _____ S1 _____ lbs S2 _____lbs S3 ____lbs

Chest Fly Machine – Do all exercises 3 sets of 8 reps. Rest 60 seconds between sets. Rest 90 seconds after completing this exercise.

Date: _____ S1 _____ lbs S2 _____lbs S3 ____lbs

Date: _____ S1 _____ lbs S2 _____lbs S3 ____lbs

Date: _____ S1 _____ lbs S2 _____lbs S3 ____lbs

Date: _____ S1 _____ lbs S2 _____lbs S3 ____lbs

Date: _____ S1 _____ lbs S2 _____lbs S3 ____lbs

Seated Rope Cable Row – Do all exercises 3 sets of 8 reps. Rest 60 seconds between sets. Rest 90 seconds after completing this exercise.

Date: _____ S1 _____ lbs S2 _____lbs S3 ____lbs

Date: _____ S1 _____ lbs S2 _____lbs S3 ____lbs

Date: _____ S1 _____ lbs S2 _____lbs S3 ____lbs

Date: _____ S1 _____ lbs S2 _____lbs S3 ____lbs

Date: _____ S1 _____ lbs S2 _____lbs S3 ____lbs

Chapter 7
Day 4

Day 4 of the "One Hour Gym" workout builds muscle mass and strength in the abs, shoulders and triceps.

Utilizing a set of 9 exercises, these three muscle groups will be worked to develop muscle mass and strength.

This series of exercises should take you less than 60 minutes to complete.

Ab Machine – Do all exercises 3 sets of 8 reps. Rest 60 seconds between sets. Rest 90 seconds after completing this exercise.

Date: _____ S1 _____ lbs S2 _____lbs S3 ____lbs

Date: _____ S1 _____ lbs S2 _____lbs S3 ____lbs

Date: _____ S1 _____ lbs S2 _____lbs S3 ____lbs

Date: _____ S1 _____ lbs S2 _____lbs S3 ____lbs

Date: _____ S1 _____ lbs S2 _____lbs S3 ____lbs

Dumbbell Arm Circles – Do all exercises 3 sets of 8 reps. Rest 60 seconds between sets. Rest 90 seconds after completing this exercise.

Date: _____ S1 _____ lbs S2 _____lbs S3 ____lbs

Date: _____ S1 _____ lbs S2 _____lbs S3 ____lbs

Date: _____ S1 _____ lbs S2 _____lbs S3 ____lbs

Date: _____ S1 _____ lbs S2 _____lbs S3 ____lbs

Date: _____ S1 _____ lbs S2 _____lbs S3 ____lbs

Dumbbell Triceps Extension, Seated – Do all exercises 3 sets of 8 reps. Rest 60 seconds between sets. Rest 90 seconds after completing this exercise.

Date: _____ S1 _____ lbs S2 _____lbs S3 ____lbs

Date: _____ S1 _____ lbs S2 _____lbs S3 ____lbs

Date: _____ S1 _____ lbs S2 _____lbs S3 ____lbs

Date: _____ S1 _____ lbs S2 _____lbs S3 ____lbs

Date: _____ S1 _____ lbs S2 _____lbs S3 ____lbs

Weighted Situps – Do all exercises 3 sets of 8 reps. Rest 60 seconds between sets. Rest 90 seconds after completing this exercise.

Date: _____ S1 _____ lbs S2 _____lbs S3 ____lbs

Date: _____ S1 _____ lbs S2 _____lbs S3 ____lbs

Date: _____ S1 _____ lbs S2 _____lbs S3 ____lbs

Date: _____ S1 _____ lbs S2 _____lbs S3 ____lbs

Date: _____ S1 _____ lbs S2 _____lbs S3 ____lbs

Shoulder Press Machine – Do all exercises 3 sets of 8 reps. Rest 60 seconds between sets. Rest 90 seconds after completing this exercise.

Date: _____ S1 _____ lbs S2 _____lbs S3 ____lbs

Date: _____ S1 _____ lbs S2 _____lbs S3 ____lbs

Date: _____ S1 _____ lbs S2 _____lbs S3 ____lbs

Date: _____ S1 _____ lbs S2 _____lbs S3 ____lbs

Date: _____ S1 _____ lbs S2 _____lbs S3 ____lbs

Dumbbell Triceps Kickback, Bench, Neutral Grip – Do all exercises 3 sets of 8 reps. Rest 60 seconds between sets. Rest 90 seconds after completing this exercise.

Date: _____ S1 _____ lbs S2 _____lbs S3 ____lbs

Date: _____ S1 _____ lbs S2 _____lbs S3 ____lbs

Date: _____ S1 _____ lbs S2 _____lbs S3 ____lbs

Date: _____ S1 _____ lbs S2 _____lbs S3 ____lbs

Date: _____ S1 _____ lbs S2 _____lbs S3 ____lbs

Torso Twist Machine – Do all exercises 3 sets of 8 reps. Rest 60 seconds between sets. Rest 90 seconds after completing this exercise.

Date: _____ S1 _____ lbs S2 _____lbs S3 ____lbs

Date: _____ S1 _____ lbs S2 _____lbs S3 ____lbs

Date: _____ S1 _____ lbs S2 _____lbs S3 ____lbs

Date: _____ S1 _____ lbs S2 _____lbs S3 ____lbs

Date: _____ S1 _____ lbs S2 _____lbs S3 ____lbs

Upright Cable Row – Do all exercises 3 sets of 8 reps. Rest 60 seconds between sets. Rest 90 seconds after completing this exercise.

Date: _____ S1 _____ lbs S2 _____lbs S3 ____lbs

Date: _____ S1 _____ lbs S2 _____lbs S3 ____lbs

Date: _____ S1 _____ lbs S2 _____lbs S3 ____lbs

Date: _____ S1 _____ lbs S2 _____lbs S3 ____lbs

Date: _____ S1 _____ lbs S2 _____lbs S3 ____lbs

Cable Triceps Push down, Overhand Grip – Do all exercises 3 sets of 8 reps. Rest 60 seconds between sets. Rest 90 seconds after completing this exercise.

Date: _____ S1 _____ lbs S2 _____lbs S3 ____lbs

Date: _____ S1 _____ lbs S2 _____lbs S3 ____lbs

Date: _____ S1 _____ lbs S2 _____lbs S3 ____lbs

Date: _____ S1 _____ lbs S2 _____lbs S3 ____lbs

Date: _____ S1 _____ lbs S2 _____lbs S3 ____lbs

Chapter 8
Day 5

Day 5 of the "One Hour Gym" workout builds muscle mass and strength in the legs, arms and back.

Utilizing a set of 9 exercises, these three muscle groups will be worked to develop muscle mass and strength.

This series of exercises should take you less than 60 minutes to complete.

Leg Press Machine – Do all exercises 3 sets of 8 reps. Rest 60 seconds between sets. Rest 90 seconds after completing this exercise.

Date: _____ S1 _____ lbs S2 _____lbs S3 ____lbs

Date: _____ S1 _____ lbs S2 _____lbs S3 ____lbs

Date: _____ S1 _____ lbs S2 _____lbs S3 ____lbs

Date: _____ S1 _____ lbs S2 _____lbs S3 ____lbs

Date: _____ S1 _____ lbs S2 _____lbs S3 ____lbs

Biceps Curl Machine – Do all exercises 3 sets of 8 reps. Rest 60 seconds between sets. Rest 90 seconds after completing this exercise.

Date: _____ S1 _____ lbs S2 _____lbs S3 ____lbs

Date: _____ S1 _____ lbs S2 _____lbs S3 ____lbs

Date: _____ S1 _____ lbs S2 _____lbs S3 ____lbs

Date: _____ S1 _____ lbs S2 _____lbs S3 ____lbs

Date: _____ S1 _____ lbs S2 _____lbs S3 ____lbs

Seated Rope Cable Row – Do all exercises 3 sets of 8 reps. Rest 60 seconds between sets. Rest 90 seconds after completing this exercise.

Date: _____ S1 _____ lbs S2 _____lbs S3 ____lbs

Date: _____ S1 _____ lbs S2 _____lbs S3 ____lbs

Date: _____ S1 _____ lbs S2 _____lbs S3 ____lbs

Date: _____ S1 _____ lbs S2 _____lbs S3 ____lbs

Date: _____ S1 _____ lbs S2 _____lbs S3 ____lbs

Hamstring Pullback Machine – Do all exercises 3 sets of 8 reps. Rest 60 seconds between sets. Rest 90 seconds after completing this exercise.

Date: _____ S1 _____ lbs S2 _____lbs S3 ____lbs

Date: _____ S1 _____ lbs S2 _____lbs S3 ____lbs

Date: _____ S1 _____ lbs S2 _____lbs S3 ____lbs

Date: _____ S1 _____ lbs S2 _____lbs S3 ____lbs

Date: _____ S1 _____ lbs S2 _____lbs S3 ____lbs

Dumbbell Biceps Curl, On Knee, Underhand Grip – Do all exercises 3 sets of 8 reps. Rest 60 seconds between sets. Rest 90 seconds after completing this exercise.

Date: _____ S1 _____ lbs S2 _____lbs S3 ____lbs

Date: _____ S1 _____ lbs S2 _____lbs S3 ____lbs

Date: _____ S1 _____ lbs S2 _____lbs S3 ____lbs

Date: _____ S1 _____ lbs S2 _____lbs S3 ____lbs

Date: _____ S1 _____ lbs S2 _____lbs S3 ____lbs

Row, Single Arm, Neutral Grip – Do all exercises 3 sets of 8 reps. Rest 60 seconds between sets. Rest 90 seconds after completing this exercise.

Date: _____ S1 _____ lbs S2 _____lbs S3 ____lbs

Date: _____ S1 _____ lbs S2 _____lbs S3 ____lbs

Date: _____ S1 _____ lbs S2 _____lbs S3 ____lbs

Date: _____ S1 _____ lbs S2 _____lbs S3 ____lbs

Date: _____ S1 _____ lbs S2 _____lbs S3 ____lbs

Abduction Machine – Do all exercises 3 sets of 8 reps. Rest 60 seconds between sets. Rest 90 seconds after completing this exercise.

Date: _____ S1 _____ lbs S2 _____lbs S3 ____lbs

Date: _____ S1 _____ lbs S2 _____lbs S3 ____lbs

Date: _____ S1 _____ lbs S2 _____lbs S3 ____lbs

Date: _____ S1 _____ lbs S2 _____lbs S3 ____lbs

Date: _____ S1 _____ lbs S2 _____lbs S3 ____lbs

Dumbbell Biceps Curl, Incline, Neutral Grip – Do all exercises 3 sets of 8 reps. Rest 60 seconds between sets. Rest 90 seconds after completing this exercise.

Date: _____ S1 _____ lbs S2 _____lbs S3 ____lbs

Date: _____ S1 _____ lbs S2 _____lbs S3 ____lbs

Date: _____ S1 _____ lbs S2 _____lbs S3 ____lbs

Date: _____ S1 _____ lbs S2 _____lbs S3 ____lbs

Date: _____ S1 _____ lbs S2 _____lbs S3 ____lbs

Dumbbell Pullover – Do all exercises 3 sets of 8 reps. Rest 60 seconds between sets. Rest 90 seconds after completing this exercise.

Date: _____ S1 _____ lbs S2 _____lbs S3 ____lbs

Date: _____ S1 _____ lbs S2 _____lbs S3 ____lbs

Date: _____ S1 _____ lbs S2 _____lbs S3 ____lbs

Date: _____ S1 _____ lbs S2 _____lbs S3 ____lbs

Date: _____ S1 _____ lbs S2 _____lbs S3 ____lbs

Chapter 9
Day 6

Day 6 of the "One Hour Gym" workout builds muscle mass and strength in the abs, triceps and chest.

Utilizing a set of 9 exercises, these three muscle groups will be worked to develop muscle mass and strength.

This series of exercises should take you less than 60 minutes to complete.

Seated Cable Crunch – Do all exercises 3 sets of 8 reps. Rest 60 seconds between sets. Rest 90 seconds after completing this exercise.

Date: _____ S1 _____ lbs S2 _____lbs S3 ____lbs

Date: _____ S1 _____ lbs S2 _____lbs S3 ____lbs

Date: _____ S1 _____ lbs S2 _____lbs S3 ____lbs

Date: _____ S1 _____ lbs S2 _____lbs S3 ____lbs

Date: _____ S1 _____ lbs S2 _____lbs S3 ____lbs

Cable Triceps Push down, Underhand Grip – Do all exercises 3 sets of 8 reps. Rest 60 seconds between sets. Rest 90 seconds after completing this exercise.

Date: _____ S1 _____ lbs S2 _____lbs S3 ____lbs

Date: _____ S1 _____ lbs S2 _____lbs S3 ____lbs

Date: _____ S1 _____ lbs S2 _____lbs S3 ____lbs

Date: _____ S1 _____ lbs S2 _____lbs S3 ____lbs

Date: _____ S1 _____ lbs S2 _____lbs S3 ____lbs

Decline Cable Fly, Single Arm – Do all exercises 3 sets of 8 reps. Rest 60 seconds between sets. Rest 90 seconds after completing this exercise.

Date: _____ S1 _____ lbs S2 _____lbs S3 ____lbs

Date: _____ S1 _____ lbs S2 _____lbs S3 ____lbs

Date: _____ S1 _____ lbs S2 _____lbs S3 ____lbs

Date: _____ S1 _____ lbs S2 _____lbs S3 ____lbs

Date: _____ S1 _____ lbs S2 _____lbs S3 ____lbs

Torso Twist Machine – Do all exercises 3 sets of 8 reps. Rest 60 seconds between sets. Rest 90 seconds after completing this exercise.

Date: _____ S1 _____ lbs S2 _____lbs S3 ____lbs

Date: _____ S1 _____ lbs S2 _____lbs S3 ____lbs

Date: _____ S1 _____ lbs S2 _____lbs S3 ____lbs

Date: _____ S1 _____ lbs S2 _____lbs S3 ____lbs

Date: _____ S1 _____ lbs S2 _____lbs S3 ____lbs

Dumbbell Triceps Extension, Behind Neck, Single Arm – Do all exercises 3 sets of 8 reps. Rest 60 seconds between sets. Rest 90 seconds after completing this exercise.

Date: _____ S1 _____ lbs S2 _____lbs S3 ____lbs

Date: _____ S1 _____ lbs S2 _____lbs S3 ____lbs

Date: _____ S1 _____ lbs S2 _____lbs S3 ____lbs

Date: _____ S1 _____ lbs S2 _____lbs S3 ____lbs

Date: _____ S1 _____ lbs S2 _____lbs S3 ____lbs

Dumbbell Bench Press, Incline, Rotating Grip – Do all exercises 3 sets of 8 reps. Rest 60 seconds between sets. Rest 90 seconds after completing this exercise.

Date: _____ S1 _____ lbs S2 _____lbs S3 ____lbs

Date: _____ S1 _____ lbs S2 _____lbs S3 ____lbs

Date: _____ S1 _____ lbs S2 _____lbs S3 ____lbs

Date: _____ S1 _____ lbs S2 _____lbs S3 ____lbs

Date: _____ S1 _____ lbs S2 _____lbs S3 ____lbs

Dumbbell Side Bend – Do all exercises 3 sets of 8 reps. Rest 60 seconds between sets. Rest 90 seconds after completing this exercise.

Date: _____ S1 _____ lbs S2 _____lbs S3 ____lbs

Date: _____ S1 _____ lbs S2 _____lbs S3 ____lbs

Date: _____ S1 _____ lbs S2 _____lbs S3 ____lbs

Date: _____ S1 _____ lbs S2 _____lbs S3 ____lbs

Date: _____ S1 _____ lbs S2 _____lbs S3 ____lbs

Dumbbell Triceps Extension, Flat Bench – Do all exercises 3 sets of 8 reps. Rest 60 seconds between sets. Rest 90 seconds after completing this exercise.

Date: _____ S1 _____ lbs S2 _____lbs S3 ____lbs

Date: _____ S1 _____ lbs S2 _____lbs S3 ____lbs

Date: _____ S1 _____ lbs S2 _____lbs S3 ____lbs

Date: _____ S1 _____ lbs S2 _____lbs S3 ____lbs

Date: _____ S1 _____ lbs S2 _____lbs S3 ____lbs

Incline Dumbbell Fly – Do all exercises 3 sets of 8 reps. Rest 60 seconds between sets. Rest 90 seconds after completing this exercise.

Date: _____ S1 _____ lbs S2 _____lbs S3 ____lbs

Date: _____ S1 _____ lbs S2 _____lbs S3 ____lbs

Date: _____ S1 _____ lbs S2 _____lbs S3 ____lbs

Date: _____ S1 _____ lbs S2 _____lbs S3 ____lbs

Date: _____ S1 _____ lbs S2 _____lbs S3 ____lbs

Chapter 10
Rest

The exercises within "One Hour Gym: 30 Day Workout" were meant to be pushed to their limits. But, muscle needs rest to recover, as well. While you participate in the "One Hour Gym: 30 Day Workout", you should also be getting plenty of sleep and fueling your body properly.

The "One Hour Gym: 30 Day Workout" is only a 6 day a week workout program so that a participant's body may have at least one day a week of recovery which is also important to proper muscle growth. It is this 'stress' and 'rest' cycle which builds maximum gains within the "One Hour Gym: 30 Day Workout".

Allow your body to have at least one day of rest from the "One Hour Gym: 30 Day Workout" per week. If you complete one 30 day cycle of the "One Hour Gym: 30 Day Workout", you can rest up to one week before starting another 30 day cycle.

Chapter 11
Repeat

Get motivated and get started back on 'Day 1'! If you think you feel the burn now, just wait until your 3rd or 4th week on the "One Hour Gym: 30 Day Workout".

After only two weeks, you should notice significant gains within muscle mass and strength. Your friends should also notice.

Continuing with "One Hour Gym: 30 Day Workout", participants see the greatest gains after one complete "One Hour Gym: 30 Day Workout" cycle. Many participants continue past a single "One Hour Gym: 30 Day Workout" cycle continuing muscle mass and strength gains through multiple consecutive 30 day cycles.

Extra Hour 1
Chest Pump

This supplemental set of the "One Hour Gym" workout builds muscle mass and strength in the Chest.

Utilizing a set of 9 exercises, this muscle group will be worked to develop muscle mass and strength.

This series of exercises should take you less than 60 minutes to complete.

Dumbbell Bench Press, Flat, Rotating Grip – Do all exercises 3 sets of 8 reps. Rest 60 seconds between sets. Rest 90 seconds after completing this exercise.

Date: _____ S1 _____ lbs S2 _____lbs S3 __ lbs

Date: _____ S1 _____ lbs S2 _____lbs S3 ____lbs

Date: _____ S1 _____ lbs S2 _____lbs S3 ____lbs

Date: _____ S1 _____ lbs S2 _____lbs S3 ____lbs

Date: _____ S1 _____ lbs S2 _____lbs S3 ____lbs

Dumbbell Bench Press, Incline, Rotating Grip – Do all exercises 3 sets of 8 reps. Rest 60 seconds between sets. Rest 90 seconds after completing this exercise.

Date: _____ S1 _____ lbs S2 _____lbs S3 ____lbs

Date: _____ S1 _____ lbs S2 _____lbs S3 ____lbs

Date: _____ S1 _____ lbs S2 _____lbs S3 ____lbs

Date: _____ S1 _____ lbs S2 _____lbs S3 ____lbs

Date: _____ S1 _____ lbs S2 _____lbs S3 ____lbs

Dumbbell Pullover – Do all exercises 3 sets of 8 reps. Rest 60 seconds between sets. Rest 90 seconds after completing this exercise.

Date: _____ S1 _____ lbs S2 _____lbs S3 ____lbs

Date: _____ S1 _____ lbs S2 _____lbs S3 ____lbs

Date: _____ S1 _____ lbs S2 _____lbs S3 ____lbs

Date: _____ S1 _____ lbs S2 _____lbs S3 ____lbs

Date: _____ S1 _____ lbs S2 _____lbs S3 ____lbs

Dumbbell Fly, Incline – Do all exercises 3 sets of 8 reps. Rest 60 seconds between sets. Rest 90 seconds after completing this exercise.

Date: _____ S1 _____ lbs S2 _____lbs S3 ____lbs

Date: _____ S1 _____ lbs S2 _____lbs S3 ____lbs

Date: _____ S1 _____ lbs S2 _____lbs S3 ____lbs

Date: _____ S1 _____ lbs S2 _____lbs S3 ____lbs

Date: _____ S1 _____ lbs S2 _____lbs S3 ____lbs

Dip Machine – Do all exercises 3 sets of 8 reps. Rest 60 seconds between sets. Rest 90 seconds after completing this exercise.

Date: _____ S1 _____ lbs S2 _____lbs S3 ____lbs

Date: _____ S1 _____ lbs S2 _____lbs S3 ____lbs

Date: _____ S1 _____ lbs S2 _____lbs S3 ____lbs

Date: _____ S1 _____ lbs S2 _____lbs S3 ____lbs

Date: _____ S1 _____ lbs S2 _____lbs S3 ____lbs

Chest Press Machine – Do all exercises 3 sets of 8 reps. Rest 60 seconds between sets. Rest 90 seconds after completing this exercise.

Date: _____ S1 _____ lbs S2 _____lbs S3 ____lbs

Date: _____ S1 _____ lbs S2 _____lbs S3 ____lbs

Date: _____ S1 _____ lbs S2 _____lbs S3 ____lbs

Date: _____ S1 _____ lbs S2 _____lbs S3 ____lbs

Date: _____ S1 _____ lbs S2 _____lbs S3 ____lbs

Chest Fly Machine – Do all exercises 3 sets of 8 reps. Rest 60 seconds between sets. Rest 90 seconds after completing this exercise.

Date: _____ S1 _____ lbs S2 _____lbs S3 ____lbs

Date: _____ S1 _____ lbs S2 _____lbs S3 ____lbs

Date: _____ S1 _____ lbs S2 _____lbs S3 ____lbs

Date: _____ S1 _____ lbs S2 _____lbs S3 ____lbs

Date: _____ S1 _____ lbs S2 _____lbs S3 ____lbs

Cable Pullover – Do all exercises 3 sets of 8 reps. Rest 60 seconds between sets. Rest 90 seconds after completing this exercise.

Date: _____ S1 _____ lbs S2 _____lbs S3 ____lbs

Date: _____ S1 _____ lbs S2 _____lbs S3 ____lbs

Date: _____ S1 _____ lbs S2 _____lbs S3 ____lbs

Date: _____ S1 _____ lbs S2 _____lbs S3 ____lbs

Date: _____ S1 _____ lbs S2 _____lbs S3 ____lbs

Cable Fly, Single Arm – Do all exercises 3 sets of 8 reps. Rest 60 seconds between sets. Rest 90 seconds after completing this exercise.

Date: _____ S1 _____ lbs S2 _____lbs S3 ____lbs

Date: _____ S1 _____ lbs S2 _____lbs S3 ____lbs

Date: _____ S1 _____ lbs S2 _____lbs S3 ____lbs

Date: _____ S1 _____ lbs S2 _____lbs S3 ____lbs

Date: _____ S1 _____ lbs S2 _____lbs S3 ____lbs

Extra Hour 2
Leg Pump

This supplemental set of the "One Hour Gym" workout builds muscle mass and strength in the Chest.

Utilizing a set of 9 exercises, this muscle group will be worked to develop muscle mass and strength.

This series of exercises should take you less than 60 minutes to complete.

Leg Raise Machine – Do all exercises 3 sets of 8 reps. Rest 60 seconds between sets. Rest 90 seconds after completing this exercise.

Date: _____ S1 _____ lbs S2 _____lbs S3 ____lbs

Date: _____ S1 _____ lbs S2 _____lbs S3 ____lbs

Date: _____ S1 _____ lbs S2 _____lbs S3 ____lbs

Date: _____ S1 _____ lbs S2 _____lbs S3 ____lbs

Date: _____ S1 _____ lbs S2 _____lbs S3 ____lbs

Calf Press Machine – Do all exercises 3 sets of 8 reps. Rest 60 seconds between sets. Rest 90 seconds after completing this exercise.

Date: _____ S1 _____ lbs S2 _____lbs S3 ____lbs

Date: _____ S1 _____ lbs S2 _____lbs S3 ____lbs

Date: _____ S1 _____ lbs S2 _____lbs S3 ____lbs

Date: _____ S1 _____ lbs S2 _____lbs S3 ____lbs

Date: _____ S1 _____ lbs S2 _____lbs S3 ____lbs

Inside Abduction Machine – Do all exercises 3 sets of 8 reps. Rest 60 seconds between sets. Rest 90 seconds after completing this exercise.

Date: _____ S1 _____ lbs S2 _____lbs S3 ____lbs

Date: _____ S1 _____ lbs S2 _____lbs S3 ____lbs

Date: _____ S1 _____ lbs S2 _____lbs S3 ____lbs

Date: _____ S1 _____ lbs S2 _____lbs S3 ____lbs

Date: _____ S1 _____ lbs S2 _____lbs S3 ____lbs

Leg Press Machine – Do all exercises 3 sets of 8 reps. Rest 60 seconds between sets. Rest 90 seconds after completing this exercise.

Date: _____ S1 _____ lbs S2 _____lbs S3 ____lbs

Date: _____ S1 _____ lbs S2 _____lbs S3 ____lbs

Date: _____ S1 _____ lbs S2 _____lbs S3 ____lbs

Date: _____ S1 _____ lbs S2 _____lbs S3 ____lbs

Date: _____ S1 _____ lbs S2 _____lbs S3 ____lbs

Hamstring Pullback Machine – Do all exercises 3 sets of 8 reps. Rest 60 seconds between sets. Rest 90 seconds after completing this exercise.

Date: _____ S1 __ _ lbs S2 _____lbs S3 ____lbs

Date: _____ S1 _____ lbs S2 _____lbs S3 ____lbs

Date: _____ S1 _____ lbs S2 _____lbs S3 ____lbs

Date: _____ S1 _____ lbs S2 _____lbs S3 ____lbs

Date: _____ S1 _____ lbs S2 _____lbs S3 ____lbs

Leg Raise Machine – Do all exercises 3 sets of 8 reps. Rest 60 seconds between sets. Rest 90 seconds after completing this exercise.

Date: _____ S1 _____ lbs S2 _____lbs S3 ____lbs

Date: _____ S1 _____ lbs S2 _____lbs S3 ____lbs

Date: _____ S1 _____ lbs S2 _____lbs S3 ____lbs

Date: _____ S1 _____ lbs S2 _____lbs S3 ____lbs

Date: _____ S1 _____ lbs S2 _____lbs S3 ____lbs

Calf Press Machine – Do all exercises 3 sets of 8 reps. Rest 60 seconds between sets. Rest 90 seconds after completing this exercise.

Date: _____ S1 _____ lbs S2 _____lbs S3 ____lbs

Date: _____ S1 _____ lbs S2 _____lbs S3 ____lbs

Date: _____ S1 _____ lbs S2 _____lbs S3 ____lbs

Date: _____ S1 _____ lbs S2 _____lbs S3 ____lbs

Date: _____ S1 _____ lbs S2 _____lbs S3 ____lbs

Outside Abduction Machine – Do all exercises 3 sets of 8 reps. Rest 60 seconds between sets. Rest 90 seconds after completing this exercise.

Date: _____ S1 _____ lbs S2 _____lbs S3 ____lbs

Date: _____ S1 _____ lbs S2 _____lbs S3 ____lbs

Date: _____ S1 _____ lbs S2 _____lbs S3 ____lbs

Date: _____ S1 _____ lbs S2 _____lbs S3 ____lbs

Date: _____ S1 _____ lbs S2 _____lbs S3 ____lbs

Leg Press Machine – Do all exercises 3 sets of 8 reps. Rest 60 seconds between sets. Rest 90 seconds after completing this exercise.

Date: _____ S1 _____ lbs S2 _____lbs S3 ____lbs

Date: _____ S1 _____ lbs S2 _____lbs S3 ____lbs

Date: _____ S1 _____ lbs S2 _____lbs S3 ____lbs

Date: _____ S1 _____ lbs S2 _____lbs S3 ____lbs

Date: _____ S1 _____ lbs S2 _____lbs S3 ____lbs

Extra Hour 3
Back Pump

This supplemental set of the "One Hour Gym" workout builds muscle mass and strength in the Back.

Utilizing a set of 9 exercises, this muscle group will be worked to develop muscle mass and strength.

This series of exercises should take you less than 60 minutes to complete.

Dumbbell Row, Single Arm, Neutral Grip – Do all exercises 3 sets of 8 reps. Rest 60 seconds between sets. Rest 90 seconds after completing this exercise.

Date: _____ S1 _____ lbs S2 _____lbs S3 ___lbs

Date: _____ S1 _____ lbs S2 _____lbs S3 ____lbs

Date: _____ S1 _____ lbs S2 _____lbs S3 ____lbs

Date: _____ S1 _____ lbs S2 _____lbs S3 ____lbs

Date: _____ S1 _____ lbs S2 _____lbs S3 ____lbs

Dumbbell Pullover – Do all exercises 3 sets of 8 reps. Rest 60 seconds between sets. Rest 90 seconds after completing this exercise.

Date: _____ S1 _____ lbs S2 _____lbs S3 ____lbs

Date: _____ S1 _____ lbs S2 _____lbs S3 ____lbs

Date: _____ S1 _____ lbs S2 _____lbs S3 ____lbs

Date: _____ S1 _____ lbs S2 _____lbs S3 ____lbs

Date: _____ S1 _____ lbs S2 _____lbs S3 ____lbs

Incline Dumbbell Pullover, Bent Arm – Do all exercises 3 sets of 8 reps. Rest 60 seconds between sets. Rest 90 seconds after completing this exercise.

Date: _____ S1 _____ lbs S2 _____lbs S3 ____lbs

Date: _____ S1 _____ lbs S2 _____lbs S3 ____lbs

Date: _____ S1 _____ lbs S2 _____lbs S3 ____lbs

Date: _____ S1 _____ lbs S2 _____lbs S3 ____lbs

Date: _____ S1 _____ lbs S2 _____lbs S3 ____lbs

Seated Rope Cable Row – Do all exercises 3 sets of 8 reps. Rest 60 seconds between sets. Rest 90 seconds after completing this exercise.

Date: _____ S1 _____ lbs S2 _____lbs S3 ____lbs

Date: _____ S1 _____ lbs S2 _____lbs S3 ____lbs

Date: _____ S1 _____ lbs S2 _____lbs S3 ____lbs

Date: _____ S1 _____ lbs S2 _____lbs S3 ____lbs

Date: _____ S1 _____ lbs S2 _____lbs S3 ____lbs

Cable Face Pull – Do all exercises 3 sets of 8 reps. Rest 60 seconds between sets. Rest 90 seconds after completing this exercise.

Date: _____ S1 _____ lbs S2 _____lbs S3 ____lbs

Date: _____ S1 _____ lbs S2 _____lbs S3 ____lbs

Date: _____ S1 _____ lbs S2 _____lbs S3 ____lbs

Date: _____ S1 _____ lbs S2 _____lbs S3 ____lbs

Date: _____ S1 _____ lbs S2 _____lbs S3 ____lbs

Cable Pullover – Do all exercises 3 sets of 8 reps. Rest 60 seconds between sets. Rest 90 seconds after completing this exercise.

Date: _____ S1 _____ lbs S2 _____lbs S3 ____lbs

Date: _____ S1 _____ lbs S2 _____lbs S3 ____lbs

Date: _____ S1 _____ lbs S2 _____lbs S3 ____lbs

Date: _____ S1 _____ lbs S2 _____lbs S3 ____lbs

Date: _____ S1 _____ lbs S2 _____lbs S3 ____lbs

Cable Lat Pull-down Row, Seated Wide Overhand Grip – Do all exercises 3 sets of 8 reps. Rest 60 seconds between sets. Rest 90 seconds after completing this exercise.

Date: _____ S1 _____ lbs S2 _____lbs S3 ____lbs

Date: _____ S1 _____ lbs S2 _____lbs S3 ____lbs

Date: _____ S1 _____ lbs S2 _____lbs S3 ____lbs

Date: _____ S1 _____ lbs S2 _____lbs S3 ____lbs

Date: _____ S1 _____ lbs S2 _____lbs S3 ____lbs

Cable Lat Pull-down Leaning Back, Narrow Overhand Grip – Do all exercises 3 sets of 8 reps. Rest 60 seconds between sets. Rest 90 seconds after completing this exercise.

Date: _____ S1 _____ lbs S2 _____lbs S3 ____lbs

Date: _____ S1 _____ lbs S2 _____lbs S3 ____lbs

Date: _____ S1 _____ lbs S2 _____lbs S3 ____lbs

Date: _____ S1 _____ lbs S2 _____lbs S3 ____lbs

Date: _____ S1 _____ lbs S2 _____lbs S3 ____lbs

Cable Lat Pull-down, Behind Neck, Wide Grip – Do all exercises 3 sets of 8 reps. Rest 60 seconds between sets. Rest 90 seconds after completing this exercise.

Date: _____ S1 _____ lbs S2 _____lbs S3 ____lbs

Date: _____ S1 _____ lbs S2 _____lbs S3 ____lbs

Date: _____ S1 _____ lbs S2 _____lbs S3 ____lbs

Date: _____ S1 _____ lbs S2 _____lbs S3 ____lbs

Date: _____ S1 _____ lbs S2 _____lbs S3 ____lbs

74

Extra Hour 4
Arm Pump

This supplemental set of the "One Hour Gym" workout builds muscle mass and strength in the Arms.

Utilizing a set of 9 exercises, this muscle group will be worked to develop muscle mass and strength.

This series of exercises should take you less than 60 minutes to complete.

Machine Biceps Curl – Do all exercises 3 sets of 8 reps. Rest 60 seconds between sets. Rest 90 seconds after completing this exercise.

Date: _____ S1 _____ lbs S2 _____lbs S3 ____lbs

Date: _____ S1 _____ lbs S2 _____lbs S3 ____lbs

Date: _____ S1 _____ lbs S2 _____lbs S3 ____lbs

Date: _____ S1 _____ lbs S2 _____lbs S3 ____lbs

Date: _____ S1 _____ lbs S2 _____lbs S3 ____lbs

Cable Biceps Curl, Seated Leaning Back – Do all exercises 3 sets of 8 reps. Rest 60 seconds between sets. Rest 90 seconds after completing this exercise.

Date: _____ S1 _____ lbs S2 _____lbs S3 ____lbs

Date: _____ S1 _____ lbs S2 _____lbs S3 ____lbs

Date: _____ S1 _____ lbs S2 _____lbs S3 ____lbs

Date: _____ S1 _____ lbs S2 _____lbs S3 ____lbs

Date: _____ S1 _____ lbs S2 _____lbs S3 ____lbs

Cable Biceps Drag Curl – Do all exercises 3 sets of 8 reps. Rest 60 seconds between sets. Rest 90 seconds after completing this exercise.

Date: _____ S1 _____ lbs S2 _____lbs S3 ____lbs

Date: _____ S1 _____ lbs S2 _____lbs S3 ____lbs

Date: _____ S1 _____ lbs S2 _____lbs S3 ____lbs

Date: _____ S1 _____ lbs S2 _____lbs S3 ____lbs

Date: _____ S1 _____ lbs S2 _____lbs S3 ____lbs

Dumbbell Biceps Curl, Standing, Underhand Grip

– Do all exercises 3 sets of 8 reps. Rest 60 seconds between sets. Rest 90 seconds after completing this exercise.

Date: _____ S1 _____ lbs S2 _____lbs S3 ____lbs

Date: _____ S1 _____ lbs S2 _____lbs S3 ____lbs

Date: _____ S1 _____ lbs S2 _____lbs S3 ____lbs

Date: _____ S1 _____ lbs S2 _____lbs S3 ____lbs

Date: _____ S1 _____ lbs S2 _____lbs S3 ____lbs

Dumbbell Biceps Curl, On Knee, Underhand Grip

– Do all exercises 3 sets of 8 reps. Rest 60 seconds between sets. Rest 90 seconds after completing this exercise.

Date: _____ S1 _____ lbs S2 _____lbs S3 ____lbs

Date: _____ S1 _____ lbs S2 _____lbs S3 ____lbs

Date: _____ S1 _____ lbs S2 _____lbs S3 ____lbs

Date: _____ S1 _____ lbs S2 _____lbs S3 ____lbs

Date: _____ S1 _____ lbs S2 _____lbs S3 ____lbs

Dumbbell Biceps Curl, Incline, Overhand Grip – Do all exercises 3 sets of 8 reps. Rest 60 seconds between sets. Rest 90 seconds after completing this exercise.

Date: _____ S1 _____ lbs S2 _____lbs S3 ____lbs

Date: _____ S1 _____ lbs S2 _____lbs S3 ____lbs

Date: _____ S1 _____ lbs S2 _____lbs S3 ____lbs

Date: _____ S1 _____ lbs S2 _____lbs S3 ____lbs

Date: _____ S1 _____ lbs S2 _____lbs S3 ____lbs

Bar Biceps Curl, Underhand Narrow Grip – Do all exercises 3 sets of 8 reps. Rest 60 seconds between sets. Rest 90 seconds after completing this exercise.

Date: _____ S1 _____ lbs S2 _____lbs S3 ____lbs

Date: _____ S1 _____ lbs S2 _____lbs S3 ____lbs

Date: _____ S1 _____ lbs S2 _____lbs S3 ____lbs

Date: _____ S1 _____ lbs S2 _____lbs S3 ____lbs

Date: _____ S1 _____ lbs S2 _____lbs S3 ____lbs

Bar Biceps Curl, Underhand Wide Grip – Do all exercises 3 sets of 8 reps. Rest 60 seconds between sets. Rest 90 seconds after completing this exercise.

Date: _____ S1 _____ lbs S2 _____lbs S3 ____lbs

Date: _____ S1 _____ lbs S2 _____lbs S3 ____lbs

Date: _____ S1 _____ lbs S2 _____lbs S3 ____lbs

Date: _____ S1 _____ lbs S2 _____lbs S3 ____lbs

Date: _____ S1 _____ lbs S2 _____lbs S3 ____lbs

Cable Biceps Curl, Overhand Grip – Do all exercises 3 sets of 8 reps. Rest 60 seconds between sets. Rest 90 seconds after completing this exercise.

Date: _____ S1 _____ lbs S2 _____lbs S3 ____lbs

Date: _____ S1 _____ lbs S2 _____lbs S3 ____lbs

Date: _____ S1 _____ lbs S2 _____lbs S3 ____lbs

Date: _____ S1 _____ lbs S2 _____lbs S3 ____lbs

Date: _____ S1 _____ lbs S2 _____lbs S3 ____lbs

Extra Hour 5
Ab Pump

This supplemental set of the "One Hour Gym" workout builds muscle mass and strength in the Abs.

Utilizing a set of 9 exercises, this muscle group will be worked to develop muscle mass and strength.

This series of exercises should take you less than 60 minutes to complete.

Weighted Situps – Do all exercises 3 sets of 8 reps. Rest 60 seconds between sets. Rest 90 seconds after completing this exercise.

Date: _____ S1 _____ lbs S2 _____lbs S3 ____lbs

Date: _____ S1 _____ lbs S2 _____lbs S3 ____lbs

Date: _____ S1 _____ lbs S2 _____lbs S3 ____lbs

Date: _____ S1 _____ lbs S2 _____lbs S3 ____lbs

Date: _____ S1 _____ lbs S2 _____lbs S3 ____lbs

Dumbbell Side Bend – Do all exercises 3 sets of 8 reps. Rest 60 seconds between sets. Rest 90 seconds after completing this exercise.

Date: _____ S1 _____ lbs S2 _____lbs S3 ____lbs

Date: _____ S1 _____ lbs S2 _____lbs S3 ____lbs

Date: _____ S1 _____ lbs S2 _____lbs S3 ____lbs

Date: _____ S1 _____ lbs S2 _____lbs S3 ____lbs

Date: _____ S1 _____ lbs S2 _____lbs S3 ____lbs

Ab Machine – Do all exercises 3 sets of 8 reps. Rest 60 seconds between sets. Rest 90 seconds after completing this exercise.

Date: _____ S1 _____ lbs S2 _____lbs S3 ____lbs

Date: _____ S1 _____ lbs S2 _____lbs S3 ____lbs

Date: _____ S1 _____ lbs S2 _____lbs S3 ____lbs

Date: _____ S1 _____ lbs S2 _____lbs S3 ____lbs

Date: _____ S1 _____ lbs S2 _____lbs S3 ____lbs

Seated Cable Crunch – Do all exercises 3 sets of 8 reps. Rest 60 seconds between sets. Rest 90 seconds after completing this exercise.

Date: _____ S1 _____ lbs S2 _____lbs S3 ____lbs

Date: _____ S1 _____ lbs S2 _____lbs S3 ____lbs

Date: _____ S1 _____ lbs S2 _____lbs S3 ____lbs

Date: _____ S1 _____ lbs S2 _____lbs S3 ____lbs

Date: _____ S1 _____ lbs S2 _____lbs S3 ____lbs

Torso Twist Machine – Do all exercises 3 sets of 8 reps. Rest 60 seconds between sets. Rest 90 seconds after completing this exercise.

Date: _____ S1 _____ lbs S2 _____lbs S3 ____lbs

Date: _____ S1 _____ lbs S2 _____lbs S3 ____lbs

Date: _____ S1 _____ lbs S2 _____lbs S3 ____lbs

Date: _____ S1 _____ lbs S2 _____lbs S3 ____lbs

Date: _____ S1 _____ lbs S2 _____lbs S3 ____lbs

Cable Side Bend – Do all exercises 3 sets of 8 reps. Rest 60 seconds between sets. Rest 90 seconds after completing this exercise.

Date: _____ S1 _____ lbs S2 _____lbs S3 ____lbs

Date: _____ S1 _____ lbs S2 _____lbs S3 ____lbs

Date: _____ S1 _____ lbs S2 _____lbs S3 ____lbs

Date: _____ S1 _____ lbs S2 _____lbs S3 ____lbs

Date: _____ S1 _____ lbs S2 _____lbs S3 ____lbs

Ab Machine – Do all exercises 3 sets of 8 reps. Rest 60 seconds between sets. Rest 90 seconds after completing this exercise.

Date: _____ S1 _____ lbs S2 _____lbs S3 ____lbs

Date: _____ S1 _____ lbs S2 _____lbs S3 ____lbs

Date: _____ S1 _____ lbs S2 _____lbs S3 ____lbs

Date: _____ S1 _____ lbs S2 _____lbs S3 ____lbs

Date: _____ S1 _____ lbs S2 _____lbs S3 ____lbs

Seated Cable Crunch – Do all exercises 3 sets of 8 reps. Rest 60 seconds between sets. Rest 90 seconds after completing this exercise.

Date: _____ S1 _____ lbs S2 _____lbs S3 ____lbs

Date: _____ S1 _____ lbs S2 _____lbs S3 ____lbs

Date: _____ S1 _____ lbs S2 _____lbs S3 ____lbs

Date: _____ S1 _____ lbs S2 _____lbs S3 ____lbs

Date: _____ S1 _____ lbs S2 _____lbs S3 ____lbs

Dumbbell Side Bend – Do all exercises 3 sets of 8 reps. Rest 60 seconds between sets. Rest 90 seconds after completing this exercise.

Date: _____ S1 _____ lbs S2 _____lbs S3 ____lbs

Date: _____ S1 _____ lbs S2 _____lbs S3 ____lbs

Date: _____ S1 _____ lbs S2 _____lbs S3 ____lbs

Date: _____ S1 _____ lbs S2 _____lbs S3 ____lbs

Date: _____ S1 _____ lbs S2 _____lbs S3 ____lbs

Keep up with
"One Hour Gym: 30 Day Workout"
for 60, 90, 120 days or more.

Discounts for multiple copies of
"One Hour Gym: 30 Day Workout"
are available at:

www.OneHourGym.com